# Lymphatic Yoga and the Water of Life

## Book 1 - "The Aquarium Within"

# LYMPHATIC YOGA

*and the*

# Water of Life

Book I - "*The Aquarium Within*"

*by Edely L. Wallace*

Printed in the United States of America

The material contained in this publication is for educational and informative use only and is not meant to be used as self diagnosis or treatment. Consult with your physician before undertaking any of the practices contained in this book.

*To my mentors*
*Andre Van Lysebeth (✝) and Dr. Fernando G. Miranda (✝)*

# $C$ontents

# Acknowledgments

This is the first book of a trilogy about Lymphatic Yoga. Subsequent books will expand on the practice and methodology of this new Yoga therapy. This book was inspired by my own journey and by my yoga students and colleagues.

I thank all those who have made my journey a joy. Special appreciation goes to Drs. Michael and Ethel Foldi for their pioneering work and continuing research in lymph therapy.

There are many people who have contributed to the completion of this book. I am grateful to all those who have supported me as I wrote the book and prepared it for publication.

My sincere thanks to Nancy Sinton and to Rachel Bowden for modeling for the pictures, to Louise Saulino, William C. Sinton II and Nancy Sinton for their tireless hours assisting in the editing process, to our photographer Aizey Pineda, and to Rachel Bowden for her amazing computer skills and great help. I also want to thank the Yogamatrix teachers, staff and family for all of their support.

*Edely L. Wallace*
*September, 2011*

# INTRODUCTION

Our hectic life can make us oblivious to the fact that our bodies are like a living aquarium. The lack of awareness of our "walking aquarium" can create almost unbearable difficulties for us. Unfortunately, we do not know what we do not know!

Our individual entities, all our cells, are bathed and nourished in this "aquarium water" that makes up the majority of the body. Like our planet, two thirds of our body is composed of water. We have different names for the various waters on the planet Earth: "ocean", "river", or "lake". Likewise, our bodily waters also have different names according to their geographic location in the body: blood, interstitial fluid, plasma, cerebrospinal fluid and lymph.

If all this water is not consistently cleaned, purified, and oxygenated, an accumulation of debris or toxins in our body is inevitable and will render the water environment poisonous to our cells - the "little fishes" in our living aquarium. Dirty, stagnant water cannot properly nourish and keep all the "little fishes"- our cells - healthy.

Bathed in this stagnant water, the "little fishes", in agony, desperately attempt to make sure we know of their difficulties. They try to get our attention by making our lives harder and, as a result, we feel discomfort and pain, followed by insomnia and diseases. They are helpless! The body's cells and tissues are gradually poisoned by the toxic water environment they live in, and organs and functions begin to deteriorate in a very slow and steady progression.

Unfortunately, most of us take these problems at face value. When diseases arise we may believe that there is a specific problem either in the liver, kidneys, stomach or intestines, for example. This may not be the entire truth. We do not know what we do not know!

As simple as it seems, the water environment just needs to be cleaned to restore cellular harmony, regulate the homeostasis of the body and ensure total health. Sadly, however, if this state of affairs continues on too long, and most of the fish or cells are dying, sorry, you have waited too long!

No need to despair! What many do not know is that it is very simple and easy to clean the water in the body-aquarium, guaranteeing a clean and healthier environment for our "little fishes", the cells.

Oxygenation is important for any aquarium and because our aquarium is very complex - like the Earth that contains many different types of rivers and streams that need to be drained - we also need a drainage system for the debris, toxins and dead cells to avoid stagnation and prevent further deterioration. The combination of both oxygenation and drainage can solve unpleasant conditions in the aquarium within.

Don't worry! There is no need for machines, external aids, or complex time-consuming practices. You just need your body, the willingness to try, and the knowledge of how to purify the liquids in the body. The knowledge, you will find in this book.

The results of this knowledge go beyond just a balanced state of health. Intangible results such as joy of life, rejuvenation, well being, and a sense of peace and balance also follow from the application of the method - Lymphatic Yoga - explained in this book.

That is what this book is about, a combination of two techniques: Yoga and Lymphatic Drainage.

Yoga is a proven method over thousands of years old, that has stood the test of time because it works. It is the only form of exercise that is truly concerned with body oxygenation, given the countless ancient breathing exercises that are included in its practice. Yoga practice restores, rejuvenates, balances and strengthens both the body and the mind.

The Lymphatic System is the fundamental "water reservoir" of the body. It holds at least twice the water of the bloodstream and bathes nearly all of the cells, tissues and organs of the body, cleansing and nourishing them. Lymphatic drainage is a more recent method that in the last decades has become well known in Europe for its effective results in cleansing, nourishing and restoring the body.

In the next chapters, you will learn about the Lymphatic System, its importance and how Yoga and the Lymphatic System match perfectly and can help each other - magnifying their unique respective benefits when combined in a single method.

# CHAPTER I

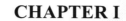

*From a Catastrophic Accident to a Book Store in Belgium*

Looking back over twenty years ago, it is amazing that my lymphatic-yoga journey started inside a bookstore in Belgium. I was browsing for yoga books as a way of health. Perhaps, I should go back in time even further and mention briefly the catastrophic accident that led me from my home town in Brazil to this little charming bookstore in Brussels.

As a busy working mom of two little girls, I was sent by my boss to take a three-week course in San Paulo, a cosmopolitan city about one hour away from my home town. "No big deal", I thought, "I can squeeze this into my schedule." I also would get a job promotion upon the course completion. My husband had recently completed his internship as a physician and some extra income would be most welcome at this time. I was happy with the upcoming promotion but also concerned about my girls and the three weeks I would not be there for them. Little did I know how much my small world was about to change forever.

On the last day of the course, after its successful completion, coming back in the winding road down to my sea shore home town, fatality struck. The bus I was riding was hit in the rear by a loaded truck and like a small toy the bus was projected off the roadway, broke through the guard rail and plunged - in a free fall of approximately 300 feet down - into the middle of the tropical forest. I was startled and really did not know what was happening.

Most people did not survive the impact of the fall. It took about three hours for the rescue crew to reach the inhospitable place where the debris of the bus were lying, along with bodies scattered on the ground for a radius of 200 meters.

To make a very long story short, I had multiple fractures including both legs, threats of leg amputation, and over the following couple of years, numerous surgeries, severe allergies, lupus, re-fractures, and all the paraphernalia that comes with this nightmare such as wheel chairs, walkers, crutches, etc.

Finally, two years after this catastrophic accident, I was told to do yoga. At this time, I had just had another leg surgery, was still bedridden and unable to move from the waistline down... I was shocked! ... How in the world I could do Yoga???

Anyway, since I could not do anything other than lie down 24 hours every day, I thought this Yoga could be a good distraction or at least a change in the scenery.

This was the way I was introduced to Yoga. Once per week the yoga teacher came to my home. As I was unable to practice physical exercises, I was instructed in breathing and relaxation techniques.  So, I practiced the breathing exercises several times per day and every day continuously.  It was simply because it was something I could do, something to occupy my long hours in bed.

Unexpectedly, at the end of about two weeks of this continuous breathing ritual, I could feel some changes!  I was astonished and doubtful.  Was it possible?  I did not have as much pain as before and my apathy or sense of helplessness decreased.  I could feel lots of energy throughout my entire body and I was even experiencing a kind of comfort and happiness.

Suddenly, I was feeling good! Something was working!  Was this the result of my breathing practice? I was clueless. I did not know.

Immediately, I decided to take my practice more seriously and began to read everything I could about what Yoga is and how it works. I wanted to know both why simple breathing techniques could make such a difference and how I could improve my breathing practice. I desperately needed to understand and to learn more!

I had a strange feeling that I could have a "bigger result." Despite gloomy medical predictions, I thought I could walk again without support and maybe this technique would be the solution. Maybe I could take care of my girls again. Maybe I could go to the school on Mother's day, or walk in the streets or simply go to the kitchen to have a glass of water. These were my dreams.

In the next few years, I engaged in a serious study, which literally took my entire days, just devouring yoga and health related books. I was practicing yoga as I could, evaluating the results on myself. I discarded what I considered not helpful and kept what I considered gems that really worked. I was steadily and slowly getting healthier and stronger while gradually knowing more, and understanding better, the Yoga method and how the body works. Finally, the "bigger result" came despite all contrary medical predictions. I could walk again!

After an odyssey of several years of obliged reclusion and lots of learning, I was finally standing by myself at the *"L'Univers Particulier"* - a specialty bookstore in Brussels. I had traveled from Brazil just to take yoga classes with Andre Van Lysebeth and learn how to teach Yoga classes from a master. In my home town, I was being asked to teach yoga. Family and friends were surprised with my unexpected recovery, youthful skin, good humor and slim body after the catastrophic accident and difficult recovery. Everybody wanted to learn more about yoga.

And there I was - standing by myself in the middle of a bookstore. It was purely exhilarating! The simple event of talking to the person at the counter, asking questions or browsing among the books, brought to me a mixed sense of incredulity and joy. It was almost a surreal situation compared to my previous condition.

I also had a feeling that there was much more to learn. I felt that I had just scratched the surface of what Yoga is and I was looking for more when I came across a "Lymphatic Drainage" book. Intrigued by the title, I grabbed the book. I had no idea what this could be about. Through my recovery experience, I came in contact or heard about diverse natural healing methods but had never heard about "lymphatic drainage".

Coincidence or not, I opened the book to a page about the therapeutic indications of lymphatic drainage for hard to heal bone fractures and how lymph drainage could work even after recurrent complications. Surprise! This was my reaction. Was this book talking to me? I did not really care, I just wanted the book and began to practice this simple type of gentle drainage on myself as soon as possible.

From this day on, many other books and short courses followed my Lymphatic System research, which finally led me - after over twenty-five years of teaching yoga and practicing lymphatic drainage on myself - to take a Lymphatic course to become a Lymph Therapist. I received this training at the leading lymphatic research center and hospital, the world-renowned "Foldi Klinic" in Germany. Now, I was ready to combine these two saving methods: Yoga and Lymph Drainage.

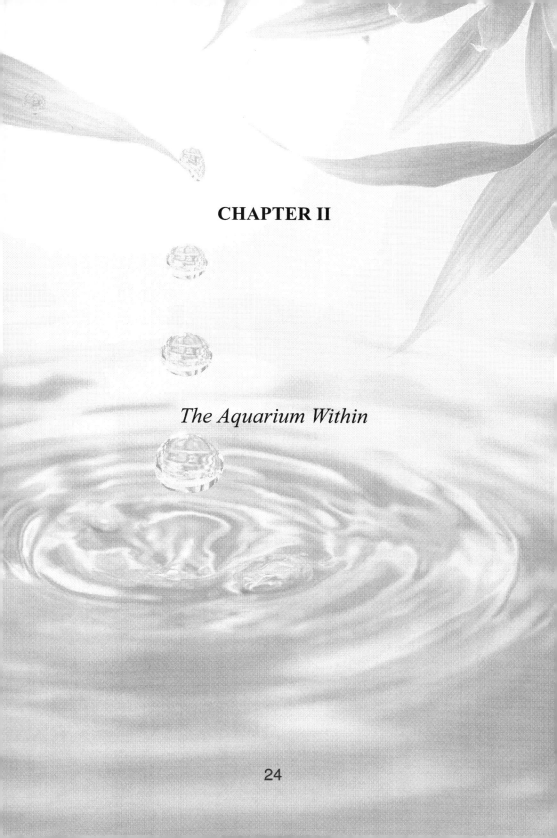

# CHAPTER II

*The Aquarium Within*

I believe my interest in lymph started earlier than the first book I purchased about lymphatic drainage. It started with my love for cooking, especially deserts. When I was grown up enough, in my early teenager years, I used to sneak into the kitchen to bake some cakes. However, my excitement about baking often created hazardous conditions in the kitchen and frequently I burned my fingers in the oven. Sure enough, a blister would appear.

The always painful blister never prevented me from wondering about the transparent water that collected so quickly in my finger. Intrigued, over and over I asked myself about the origin of this liquid. Of course, I was wounded. But, why was there no blood there? Where could this water be possibly coming from?

Well, now I know that this water is the lymph. All cells of the body are bathed in this water. In fact, the blood is unable to nourish the

25

cells because it does not come in direct contact with them. The lymph does.

The lymph originally is the plasma that leaks from the blood capillaries, bathes the cells - as interstitial liquid - and is then collected by the lymphatic capillaries to return to the heart and blood circulation. This fluid, when collected by the lymphatic capillaries, is named lymph. So, lymph, plasma and interstitial liquid are basically the same fluid, which merely receives different names depending on its location in the body.

Evolutionarily speaking, the origin of the Lymphatic System goes back to the transition of life from water to land in the beginnings of time. For instance, fish possess neither lymph vessels nor lymph nodes (1). One of the tasks of the lymphatic vessels is to absorb fatty acids and it is proved that fish absorb fatty acids in their blood systems (1).

The Lymphatic System clearly appeared first in frogs (amphibians). Curiously, frogs do not drink water, they absorb water through their skin into a network of lymph vessels that are contained in "lymph sacs" (1). So, researchers came to believe that the lymph vessels are an internal manifestation that appeared as a response to the loss of the surrounding environmental water (1). **The lymph fluid, then became the "living water", which supports our bodies in the same way that water supported life in the beginning of time.**

The Lymphatic System became the water reservoir - the "aquarium within". In other words, the water that was present in the first stages of life development moved from the outside of the body to the inside and created the Lymphatic System. The body becomes an aquarium with gallons of lukewarm seawater with trillions of cells, like fish that are bathed and nourished in this living water.

The word lymph comes from the Latin "limpidus" which means clear or limpid. Hippocrates, the father of Medicine, called it the "white blood." The Renaissance period led to a renewed interest in the Lymphatic System and some new discoveries emerged. However, it was only in 1876 that the anatomist Sappey published "Atlas", the first lymph map of the human body which is still in use today. Though a road map to the lymph was available, there was no clear understanding of the lymphatic functions at this time.

It was not until 1894, when the Starling Law of Filtration and Reabsorption explained the mechanism that allows liquid to be exchanged between blood and tissue. It all happens at the micro level. It is based on a play of different pressures exerted by the fluid inside and outside the capillaries.

The lymph gained relevance in 1912, with Nobel Prize winner Alexis Carrel, the father of modern organ transplant. One of his experiments demonstrated that chicken cells bathed in lymph liquid that was continuously renewed could live many years longer than the expected life of a chicken (2).

Impressed by this experiment, which was widely publicized in the news, the Dane, Dr. Emil Vodder developed a manual method to drain the lymph in 1932. Based on gentle massage he designed precise hand strokes to prevent stagnation of metabolic wastes and keep the bodily fluids continuously moving and renewed. His method was not immediately recognized by the medical community.

In the sixties Foldi, Asdonk, Casley-Smith and other physicians and researchers aware of the positive results of Dr. Vodder's lymphatic drainage method, began to clinically test his method. In 1967, Johannes Asdonk, a German physician, conducted research on 20,000 patients. He established the medical effects and indications and contraindications of manual lymph drainage.

Physicians Michael Foldi and his wife Ethel Foldi, after years of research, combined the lymph drainage concepts of Dr. Vodder with other therapies. During the 1980s, the Foldi's created the "Complex Decongestive Therapy", which today is widely used in the treatment of lymphedema.

In 1986, they opened the renowned "Foldi Clinic" in Germany to treat patients with lymphedema and lymph related diseases. In 1995, the International Society of Lymphology endorsed Foldi's method as the most effective therapy for lymphedema. Today, the "Foldi Clinic" accepts lymphedema patients from all over the world. "Foldi's Textbook of Lymphology" is considered the Lymphatic System *bible* for physicians and therapists.

# CHAPTER III

*The Cinderella System of the Body -*
*The Lymphatic System*

Throughout the recovery period, forcibly in bed and practicing Yoga in my spare time - that means all the time, in one form or another - I also learned how important it is to know how the body and its systems work in detail.

As I discovered the oddities of the body, rather than a tedious task, this study became a fascinating journey. To learn the complexities of the body and how every tissue and organ can affect each other in unsuspected ways led me to better application and better results of my yoga practice. I had realized that what I did not know could hurt me!

Likewise, the knowledge of the landscape of the Lymphatic System does not disappoint in terms of the practical application that can be extracted from it in order to improve, maintain, rejuvenate or restore the body.

## HOW IMPORTANT IS THE LYMPH?

Decades ago, the Harvard Medical School researcher, Cecil Drinker, prophesied that *"the Lymphatic System is the most important vital system of men and animals"*. Today, the Lymphatic System probably is the least known bodily system among the general public.

Probably, because nobody specifically dies of a "lymphatic attack", the humble Lymphatic System has gone unnoticed until now.

We all know that the body is mainly water - about 70-75%. Blood comprises about 20% of this bodily water. Fewer people know that there is another system in the body that holds at least twice as much water as the bloodstream.

The Lymphatic System is the body's fundamental water reservoir. It bathes all cells, tissues and organs of the body, cleansing and nourishing them. It also is the transport and drainage system of the body. Our "aquarium within" relies on the Lymphatic System for cell renewal, tissue repair and cell nutrition. The Lymphatic System is so vital to all structures of the body that its condition can be considered the "mirror of our health".

Strictly speaking, the Lymphatic System cannot be labeled as a circulatory system because it is a one-way system. It flows towards the heart. Lymph vessels begin in the periphery and end near the heart into the venous circulatory system through the venous angle behind the collarbone (3).

Unlike the Cardiovascular System which relies on the heart to pump the blood, the Lymphatic System does not have a central pump to assist its flow. So, **the lymph is a slow system by nature, one that mainly moves because of muscle activity and deep breathing.**

The Lymphatic System is mainly composed of lymph, lymphatic vessels and lymphatic nodes. Necessarily brief but fundamental information about the lymph system follows:

# LYMPH

The lymph is a transparent or whitish liquid derived from the interstitial fluid. The lymph fluid - the "aquarium water" of the body - is composed of 96% water (4) and permeates nearly all structures and bathes all cells of the body. **The lymph carries vital nutrients to the cells, it receives their metabolic waste and transports their waste to the heart**.

Besides water the lymph fluid is also composed of protein molecules, fatty acids, minerals, vitamins, lymphocytes, enzymes, dead cells, toxins, debris, dust, bacteria, virus, cancer cells and gases. The lymph content is known as "lymphatic load", as termed by German researcher Dr. Foldi.

Because protein molecules are continuously leaking from the bloodstream into the interstitial fluid, it is vital that they return to the blood. As proteins leave the bloodstream they carry with them "little gifts". Proteins are the vehicle for vitamins, hormones, minerals to be delivered to the cells (5).

It is important to know that throughout a single day more than half the protein content of the blood leaks from the bloodstream. If the protein does not return to the blood in 24 hours, a "fatal hypovolemic shock occurs" or death is the result (6). So, **the transport of the protein back to the bloodstream is considered the most important function of the Lymphatic System** (6).


## LYMPHATIC VESSELS - *Little Hearts*

In its journey back to the bloodstream the lymph enters the initial lymph vessels (lymph capillaries) which are larger than the blood capillaries. Their main function is to collect the interstitial fluid. Like a net, the valveless lymph capillaries cover the entire surface of the body (7).

The heart is the destination of the lymph fluid. Progressively, the lymph moves from capillaries to larger lymph vessels, known as pre-collectors, to collectors, trunks, and ducts.

The lymph collectors are both larger and more complex vessels than the capillaries. They are built from valved segments with "muscular units"(8).

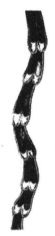

These valves are known as *lymphangions* and they "have an extensive innervation" from the autonomic nervous system(8). *Lymphangions* also have an intrinsic motion, they pulsate like "little hearts" to help to pump the lymph (9). They give direction to the lymph and prevent lymph backflow (10).

**Stress directly affects lymphangions' pumping function because of their "extensive innervation" and close connection with the Nervous System. Stress is one of the causes of lymph stagnation.**

The largest lymphatic vessels are the lymph trunks, which exit into the venous circulation close to the heart. The largest lymph trunk is the *thoracic duct*. It is about 2 to 5 mm in diameter and 40 cm long. It parallels the spine from the lumbar spine to the base of the neck. It originates below the diaphragm as a sac-like enlargement named *cisterna chyli* (11).

In its trajectory the lymph flow passes through one or more filtering stations - the lymphatic nodes.

## LYMPHATIC NODES

When a tooth infection occurs we may feel the jaw and neck areas both swollen and sore. Or, when we have a cut toe or an infected toe nail, we may feel soreness in the groin area. These are the lymphatic nodes doing their work.

The nodes are like sentinel stations that filter, clean and immunologically boost the lymph that moves through them. Lymph nodes retain, neutralize and break down toxins, bacteria and viruses as they produce antibodies known as lymphocytes.

There are about 600-700 lymph nodes (12). Usually, they occur in clusters spread throughout the body (12). The neck and abdominal area contain a great number of the lymph nodes. Other lymph nodes are spread throughout the body, especially in the joints.(13)

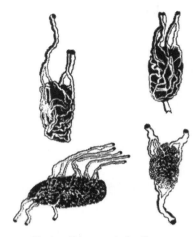

Besides filtering and cleansing the lymph, the nodes produce lymphocytes to fight diseases. They also regulate the concentration of protein in the lymph (14). The lymph flow is slowed down by the filtering and cleansing functions of lymph nodes.

*Traite d'Anatomie by Sappey*

Throughout the course of life, lymph nodes and the Lymphatic System go to involution. Age related involution affects the center part of the nodes, though, their outer edges remain intact, like a shell. It is proved that active organs undergo less degeneration (15).

## LYMPHATIC SYSTEM FUNCTIONS

This neglected system can rightly be called the "Cinderella System" of the body.

It humbly cleans the trash of all other systems while it feeds them with nutrients such as proteins, vitamins and minerals. It carefully filters and destroys bacteria and toxins; efficiently collects and returns protein and water to the heart; diligently absorbs fat and vigilantly recognizes and responds to microbes, foreign and cancer cells. Finally, the Lymphatic System bravely fights disease and infection by producing lymphocytes.

**The *Lymphatic System* is the septic system, the defense and also the nourisher of the body.** It is the "Cinderella System" , waiting to be fully recognized as one of the most crucial and important systems of the body.

## SLUGGISH LYMPH

Since the lymph is naturally slowed down when it reaches the lymphatic nodes, any additional slowing down factor may retard the lymph to almost unbearable or even fatal levels. Sedentary life, poor breathing, stress, diseases, accidents, aging and surgeries contribute to slowing it down even further and the lymph gets sluggish.

Sluggish lymph cannot work efficiently and gradually becomes stagnant as it retains toxins, debris, and dead cells. Sluggish lymph is unable to properly nourish the tissues. The lymph nodes become overloaded with the buildup of debris, which further slows down the lymph. The lymph rich protein content is unable to move, and it hardens, generating fibrotic tissues, calcification and necrosis over time. The production of lymphocytes and the immune response is impaired.

Help! The body is in chaos! The clean water of the aquarium within, now is dirty and cannot accomplish its functions. All the trash normally filtered out and destroyed by the lymph is now thrown into other organs. The body cells and tissues are gradually poisoned by the toxic water environment they live in, and they begin to age and deteriorate slowly.

**It is important to understand that the lymph fluid must be cleaned, purified and renewed like the water of an aquarium. It is also important to remember that the lymph is activated by breathing and body motion. It is essential that physical exercises along with proper breathing exercises are practiced regularly to prevent lymph stagnation.**

## LYMPHATIC YOGA

The ancient Yoga method becomes the ideal way to activate and renew the lymph fluid. A combination of breathing techniques and specific Yoga postures - focused on the anatomy of the Lymphatic System - can assure both the oxygenation of the body and the drainage of the toxins guaranteeing a clean and healthier environment for our little "fishes", the cells.

A Lymphatic Yoga practice can prevent catastrophic conditions in the body while it regenerates the tissues and boosts the immune system. It also improves nutritional absorption and the general condition of all tissues and organs. It strengthens the immune system by increasing the number of lymphocytes - the antibodies - that circulate in the lymph and blood. Practicing Lymphatic Yoga also provides a relaxed state and a feel-good sensation because the Lymph System is directly related to the parasympathetic nervous system. As a result, a quiet mind and a state of peaceful joy emerge naturally.

It is important to become aware of the paramount importance of our "aquarium within", along with simple ways to cleanse and drain our "water of life", which is essential for cell renewal, tissue repair and cell nutrition. However, again, **probably because nobody specifically dies of a "lymphatic attack", the humble Lymphatic System has gone unnoticed until now.** The Lymphatic System is so vital to all structures of the body that its condition can be considered the mirror of our health.

*All pictures in this chapter are from "Traite d'Anatomie Descriptive" by Sappey (1886)*

*Traite d'Anatomie by Sappey*

*Lymphnodes and Lymph Vessels*

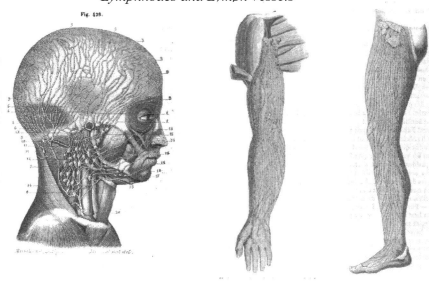

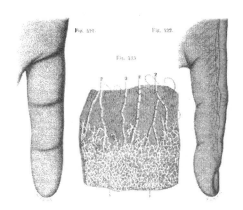

# CHAPTER IV

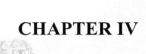

*The Ebb and Flow of the Aquarium - The Breath*

*"A yogi measures the span of life by the number of breaths, not by the number of years."*
*Swami Sivananda*

When I went to Belgium to study with the renowned Yoga master and author Andre Van Lysebeth, I already had a good grasp of his work through his books. They had helped me in ways I cannot even describe and I wanted to learn how to be a Yoga teacher from him.

Andre was one of the pioneers of Yoga in the Western world. He was the one that opened the way for Yoga to become known and available to the public everywhere. In the 1960s, the accomplished Yoga master and physician Swami Sivananda, asked Andre to create a Yoga magazine for European dissemination. For over 40 years he wrote and published the first European Yoga magazine without missing a beat of it and sometimes to the detriment of his own printing business.

One of the many things I learned from him was the importance of the breath and how to breathe correctly. Besides all of the vital benefits proper breathing brings to our multicellular being, the breathing function also is one of the main pumps of the Lymphatic System. So, it is vital to learn the essentials of this noble bodily function.

Consistently, Yoga method makes us remember that air and oxygen are the most important nutrition for the body. But, who cares? We are all more concerned with the food we eat rather than the air we breathe. However, all functions of the body need oxygen to perform their tasks. Digestion, for instance, is a complex biochemical function that relies on the levels of oxygenation of the body to be accomplished.

Poor breathing translates into impaired digestion and poor assimilation. Over time, poor assimilation leads to diseases. It is important to remember we can survive without food or water for some days, but we cannot survive without air for more than a few minutes. But, who cares?

There is a Yoga concept that says: **life and breath are the same.** Life comes with the first inhalation. Life goes with the last exhalation. And life is sustained by a series of breaths. So, according to this idea, the way we breathe directly affects conditions not only in our body but also in our daily life. But, who cares?

Well, we should care.

Usually, when asked to breathe deeply, people lift their chests. Really? Instead, they should be thinking about the diaphragm and moving their belly area. The diaphragm is the muscle in charge of 75% of the inhalation. The diaphragm is below the lungs. Over the years we all distort the breathing pattern without noticing it. It is almost as though we put the diaphragm in retirement and the breathing becomes a shallow, superficial and poor bodily activity.

Yoga considers aging more as a disease than an inevitable fatality. The breathing capacity, its depth and rhythm has a lot to do with this yogic idea. Newborns breathe diaphragmatically. If you could see a newborn sleeping you would see that they move only the belly. This is our natural breathing.

However, because of tight clothing, belts, life-stress and other factors, gradually the breathing becomes distorted. Also observe your dog or cat when they are sleeping and notice the movement of their bellies. Dogs and cats breathe properly.

The upper and middle part of the lungs are much smaller than the lower part. So, when we breathe shallowly, in the upper or middle part of the lungs, we deprive our body and mind of vital energy. We deprive ourselves of oxygen! Consequently, the body suffers, the mind gets agitated, confused (and sometimes dumb!) and stress sets in. All, pure lack of oxygenation!

On the other hand, regular, deep diaphragmatic breathing is the key to calmness, vitality and a clear mind. The deep, steady and slow motion of the diaphragmatic breathing becomes like a wave that washes the body in an unceasing ebb and flow, a wave that cradles, nourishes and imprints a particular rhythm to all living beings.

The ebb and flow of the proper breathing perhaps reestablishes the rhythm of the ocean from primordial time. It imprints a natural rhythm to the "aquarium within" that can be very soothing and healing.

To return to our baby breath and restore the correct breathing pattern, we have to become aware of simple elements of respiratory physiology:

1) the lungs cannot draw air inside themselves. They are like two inert, passive and elastic sponges.

2) it is the muscles around the lungs that move the air inside and outside the lungs by a process of expansion and contraction,

3) the major muscle involved in the breathing process is the diaphragm, a large dome-like muscle that separates the chest from the abdomen. The diaphragm is below the lungs.

4) the nose, rather than the mouth, is the correct organ for inhalation. Among other functions, the nose filters, humidifies and warms the air.

Basically, when we inhale properly, the diaphragm moves down and pushes the abdominal area forward; when we exhale, the diaphragm moves up, squeezes the residual air from the lungs, and the abdomen returns. The up and down motion of the diaphragm also provides a natural massage for internal organs (for pictures and practice see p. 71).

During the inhalation, the diaphragm squeezes the stagnated blood from the viscera; during exhalation it releases the viscera and allows fresher blood to come in. This motion revitalizes and restores functions of such organs as the liver, kidneys, pancreas, adrenal glands, gall bladder, spleen and intestines.

The proper breathing becomes a conscious act that ideally should be deep, slow and steady. The lungs need time for the exchange of oxygen and carbon dioxide to be maximized.

The up and down motion of the "muscle of life" - the diaphragm - also activates the lymphatic nodes and vessels in the abdominal area. The motion of the diaphragm helps the lymphatic inflow into the largest lymph trunk - *the thoracic duct*. It creates a suction effect in the *cisterna chyli (chapter III),* which helps lymph transport and improves cell nourishment, tissue repair and immune response in our multicellular being.

The final destination of the lymph is the heart. The heart pumps the mixed venous blood and lymph - sorry, now called plasma - to the lungs. The lungs oxygenate and purify this incoming stream in direct proportion to the amount of oxygen present in their alveoli. These are the tiny sacs where the "magical" exchange of carbon dioxide and oxygen happens inside the lungs for life to go on.

Now, the renewed plasma returns to the heart and arterial flow only to exude again from the blood capillaries - as lymph fluid - to nourish all the cells of the aquarium within.

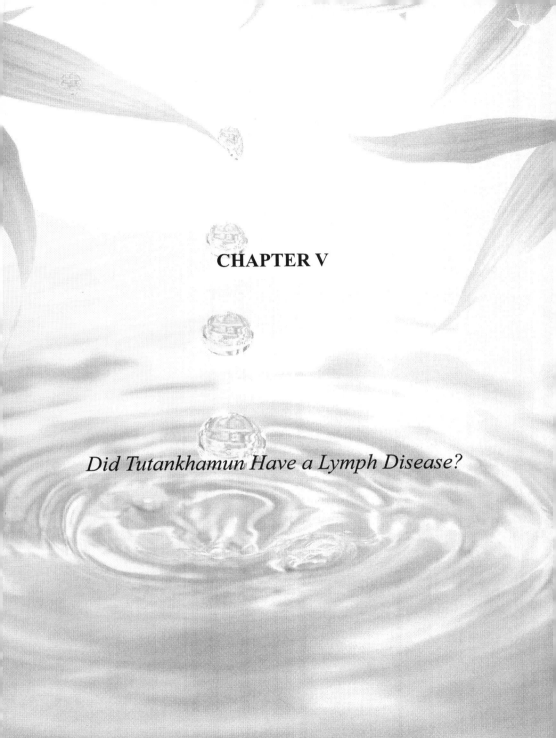

# CHAPTER V

*Did Tutankhamun Have a Lymph Disease?*

Having a degree in Philosophy makes you wonder about strange things. Fascinated by ancient Egyptian history, I sometimes asked myself about Pharaoh Tuthankamon's - *King Tut* - possible disease.

The legendary *King Tut* ascended to the throne at age 9 and died young at 19 in 1323 B.C. in Egypt. He was buried with canes and medicines, besides a myriad of treasures, according to archeological findings. In some drawings he is also depicted using a cane.

Archeologists believe he had some type of disease but do not know which disease plagued him. In 2010, in the first DNA study conducted on Egyptian royal mummies, a team of researchers examined *King Tut's* body and "revealed a previously unknown deformation" in his foot. He also had necrosis or bone tissue death in his left foot.(18)

Research has proved inconclusive regarding the disease that led to his death - he also had malaria. They hypothesized that he could have had a congenital malformation or disease caused by inbreeding, since his parents were siblings.

It is possible that *King Tut* had congenital lymphedema. It is possible he was born with a malformation of the lymphatic system - some lymph nodes absent, for instance. This would lead to lymphedema, which causes edema and a progressive accumulation and stagnation of lymph fluid. Because the lymph fluid is rich in protein, if the lymphedema is untreated the protein will harden. This leads to fibrotic tissues, calcification and necrosis or death of the tissues.

Lymphedema is an abnormal accumulation of protein-rich fluid in the interstitial spaces that usually causes chronic inflammation and reactive fibrosis of the affected area (16). As an analogy, if an unfinished yogurt container is left in the sink, the yogurt will quickly harden because it is rich in protein. The same happens in the body. If the lymph is stagnant it will also harden. Over time, this may lead to lymphedema.

Lymphedema can be divided in two types: primary (congenital) or secondary (acquired). Congenital lymphedema usually manifests very early in infancy, childhood or in puberty.

Secondary lymphedema, the most common manifestation can be caused by: cancer, surgery and/or radiation for cancer, trauma, infection, chronic venous insufficiency, obesity, mosquito bite (filariasis), air travel (Casley-Smith, 1996) (16), reduced protein intake can also lead to lymph disturbance. Filariasis is caused by a parasite, it is rare in the US and more common in underdeveloped countries.

Lymphedema is not contagious and affects about 3 million Americans. It is a common progressive disease that can become a serious one, if untreated. Lymphedema usually affects arms, legs, head and neck, intestines and genitals (16).

Lymphedema is a chronic and incurable disease that requires weekly continuous care such as manual lymph drainage, bandaging, special garments, skin care, and an exercise program (17).

**Lymphedema Signs**

- Discomfort - heaviness, pain sensation
- Onset may be slow or rapid
- Progressive
- Cellulite is common
- Often starts in the extremities
- Skin changes in the later stages

Edema is not considered lymphedema but can be a precursor to lymphedema when edema becomes repetitive and over the years becomes worse. **There are four stages in Lymphedema** (17):

- Stage O - Latency or subclinical stage
- Stage 1 - Reversible - pitting and swelling retains the indentation
- Stage 2 - Spontaneously irreversible - fluid accumulation and fibrosis
- Stage 3 - Elephantiasis - hardening of tissues, scar tissue

In the US, the highest incidence of lymphedema is found among those who have had breast cancer surgery, specifically those with lymph node removal and radiation therapy. Lymphedema can be prevented if timely remedial measures are taken after surgery or radiation.

At the "Foldi Clinic", after breast cancer surgery and removal of lymph nodes, the therapy used is to manually reroute the lymph fluid to healthy lymph nodes. This occurs through the anastomoses or alternative collateral circulation of the Lymphatic System.

The lymph can be redirected to the nodes or vessels that were not removed or irradiated and to the areas of the Lymphatic System that are still healthy. After a series of treatments, these new lymphatic routes are established. A self-care treatment is taught to the patient for self-maintenance. This therapy is not readily available in the US.

Lymphedema after breast cancer surgery, lymph node dissection or radiation, is preventable. Armed with the right information and correct techniques lymphedema should not be feared, as it can and should be avoided.

# CHAPTER VI

*It is All About Practice*

Now, it is all about practice!

The accomplished yoga master Sivananda once said: *"an ounce of practice is worth several tons of theory."* That means that theory is relatively nothing and all this knowledge becomes useless, if not applied. We must apply the information to get the results.

For instance, when you have a headache, somebody shares with you how easily you can get rid of it by taking aspirin. Excited about the new discovery (supposing you came from another planet and did not know about aspirins), you talk about it to all your family and you call friends to share the good news. However, without taking the medicine, you just talk about it. Only the knowledge of the benefits of aspirin will do nothing for your headache. You have to take the medicine. Now, it is time to put in practice the information about the Lymphatic System.

Before the practice, there are simple daily steps you can take to improve lymph transport:

- drink lots of water
- walk
- reduce salt intake in the diet
- avoid restrictive clothing that compresses the lymphatic nodes
- gently brush the body with movements towards the heart
- drink purified or filtered water
- avoid processed foods
- engage in a nutritional detox method
- swim or walk in water
- take a deep and slow breath often
- drink a glass of hot water with lemon when waking up

**General Guidelines for the practice**

First thing in the morning, before breakfast, is the best time for the practice - it prepares you for the day. Make sure you wear loose and comfortable clothing. In your practice room, try to have some fresh air or practice outside, on the terrace or in the garden.

The Yoga positions are called "asanas", which literally means "steady and comfortable pose". So, it is important not to force. **Do less then what you can do** - this is the way to progress quickly in Yoga. Do not hurry the poses. Do the motions consciously and slowly. Combine each exercise with deep abdominal breathing.

✹ Asanas are not forced exercises. Both awareness of what you are doing as you do it and the proper breathing are the foundations of success in the Yoga practice.
✹ If you are short on time, rather than hurrying the pace of the exercises, reduce the number of the poses.
✹ Avoid contracting muscles that are not maintaining the pose. Relax the muscles that are not involved in the pose.
✹ Slowly undo the pose, reversing the way you went into it.
✹ The conscious pace of the practice is essential for the effectiveness of the practice.
✹ Always end the practice with the resting pose (*shavasana*) for at least five minutes.

**Try to practice in the order prescribed. In the beginning there are warm-ups (repetitive motions). If you are new to exercising and any one of the asanas is not comfortable or within your scope, do not worry! First, practice only the easiest motions in the order prescribed. After you get stronger and more supple, gradually try the more difficult motions without pain or forcing.**

# LYMPHATIC YOGA PRACTICE

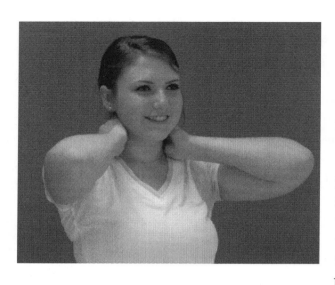

## 1.Neck Massage

Place your hands at the back of the neck and gently press and release the neck area a few times. As you do this gentle massage bring the attention to the neck and use the right pressure, avoid forcing or straining. Be gentle with yourself. Slowly, breathe in and out through the nose. After that, also press and release the area between neck and shoulders.

## 2. Neck Motions

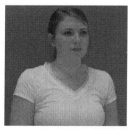 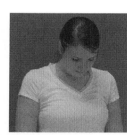 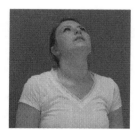

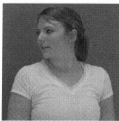 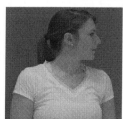

Start with your head facing forward and chin parallel to the ground. Exhale, tuck your chin slightly in and bring it toward your chest. Inhale and slowly lift the chin toward the ceiling. Synchronize breath and motion. Exhale, bring your chin down to the chest; inhale, back to center, head facing forward. Exhale and slowly rotate the head to the right, look over the shoulder. Inhale, bring the head back to center. Exhale and slowly rotate the head to the left looking over the left shoulder. Inhale, back to center. Exhale and slowly lower your right ear toward your right shoulder, chin in slightly. Inhale, bring your head back to center. Exhale and bring your left ear toward your left shoulder, chin in slightly. Exhale and bring your head back to center. Repeat all twice more.

## 3. Shoulder Dragging

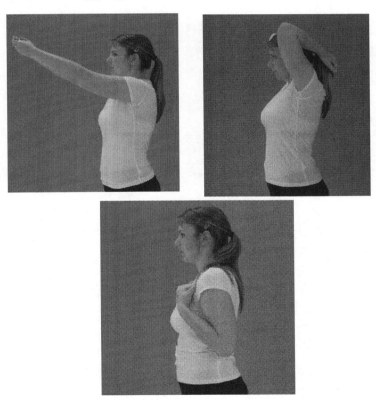

Inhale, raise both arms up and bring your hands between the shoulder blades. Gently press your hands. Exhale, keep a continuous pressure and drag both hands forward across the shoulders and collar bones. Finish by shaking the hands out. Repeat the motion 3 to 5 times.


## 4. Shoulder Lift

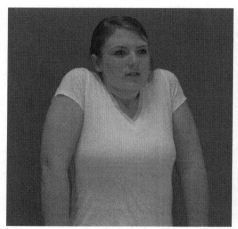 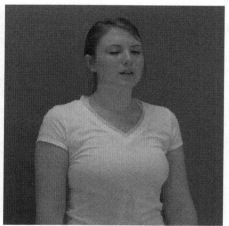

Both arms relaxed along side the torso. Inhale and slowly lift both shoulders up towards your ears. Exhale with a sigh as you drop both shoulders - let them go. Allow your arms to relax back along your sides. Repeat several times. Lift the shoulders, without forcing, a little bit higher each time.

## 5. Elbow Circles

Bend both elbows and reach them out to your sides. Relax your fingers on the top of your shoulders. Bring the attention to the elbows and draw circles in the air with both elbows, creating a rotation at the shoulders. First

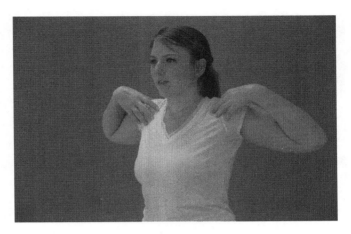

go in a backward direction several times and then pause and go in a forward direction several times.

## 6. Marching in Place

Stand facing forward with both arms relaxed along your sides. Lift the left knee and tap the left thigh with the left hand. Lower the left leg. Repeat on the other side. Continue the motion alternately, as you march in place. Relax the face, relax the arm that is not working and avoid holding the breath.

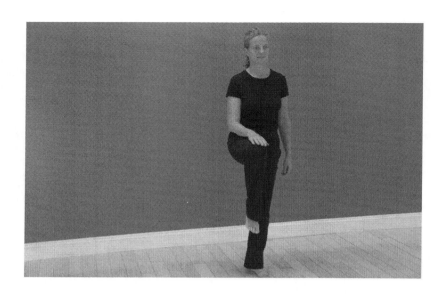

## 7. Marching in Place with Crossover

Stand with both arms relaxed along the sides. Lift your left knee and bring your bent right elbow towards this knee. Lower the left leg. Repeat on the other side. Continue the motion as you march in place alternating left knee and right elbow closer to each other and vice-versa.

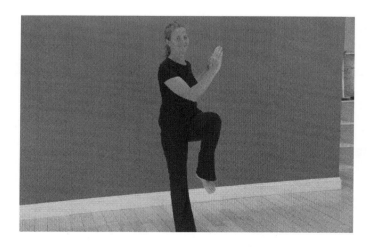

## 8. Arm Lift - Heels Up - Chin up

a) Stand with feet shoulder width apart and head facing forward. Chin parallel to the ground. Both arms relaxed along side. Long inhalation as you slowly raise both arms out to the sides and up overhead. Relax your shoulders. Exhale and slowly lower both arms. Synchronize breath and motion. Repeat twice.

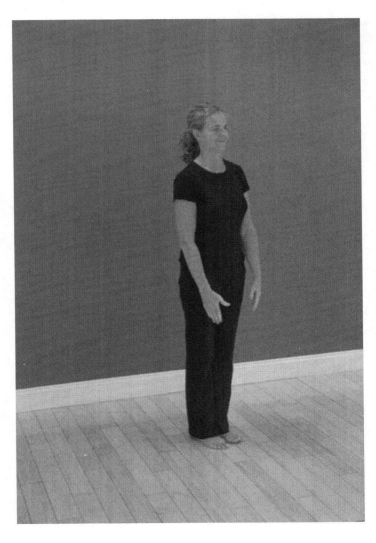

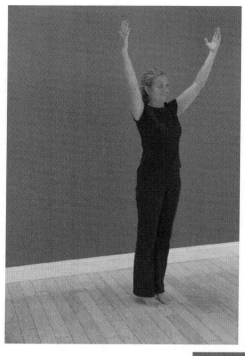

b)Inhale and simultaneously, raise both arms and heels to come up onto the balls of the feet. Exhale and slowly lower arms as you lower the heels back to the ground. Repeat twice.

c) Inhale and slowly raise both arms, simultaneously, lift both heels as you come

up onto the balls of the feet and gradually look up as you point the chin toward the ceiling. As you exhale, simultaneously and slowly lower arms and heels and bring your chin slightly in and toward the chest. Look toward your heart. Repeat twice. Breathe deeply and slowly. Finish with the heels on the ground, arms by your side and head facing forward.

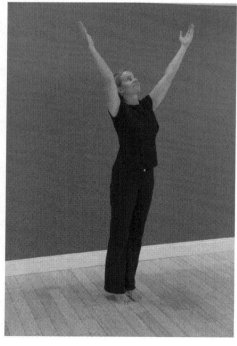

## 9. Half Moon

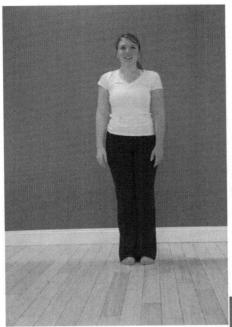

Stand with feet together. Inhale as you lift the right arm over head. Squeeze your buttocks and lean your trunk to the left, as you exhale. As you inhale press your right foot on the floor; as you exhale relax your trunk to left a little more and only what is comfortably possible. Stay into the pose for three long breaths.

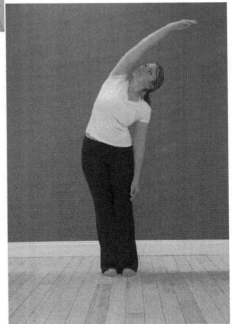

Every time you inhale, mentally observe your ribs separating on the right side.
As you exhale, notice the ribs returning. At the end, inhale and centralize the spine; exhale and lower the right arm. Repeat on the other side.

## 10. Ankle Movements / Leg Squeeze

Sit with both legs stretched out and together in front of you. Exhale and point your feet away from you, inhale and flex your feet towards you. Repeat several times. Stop the motion. Circle both ankles together several times in one direction and then pause and circle them in the other direction. Stop the motion. Inhale and gradually squeeze the muscles of the legs starting with the buttocks, then the thighs, then the knees and calves. Exhale and relax all. Repeat this squeezing and releasing four times. On your last set hold the squeeze for three breaths - every time you inhale, squeeze a little more thighs, knees and calves - then, release as you exhale.

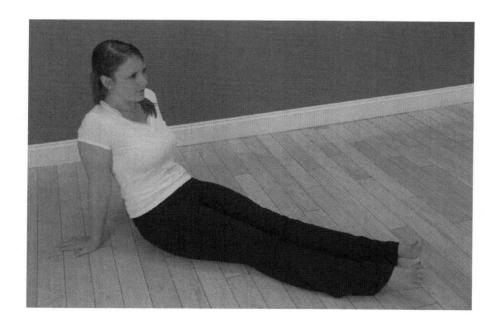

## 11. Lying Down - Knees Together, Feet Apart / Vice-versa

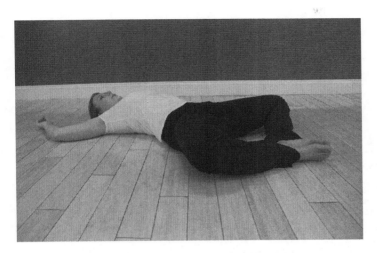

Lie down on your back with your knees bent. Arms relaxed over the head, on the floor. Inhale and separate your knees out to the sides and toward the floor as you bring the soles of the feet together. Exhale, bring the knees together and feet apart. Repeat the motion several times.

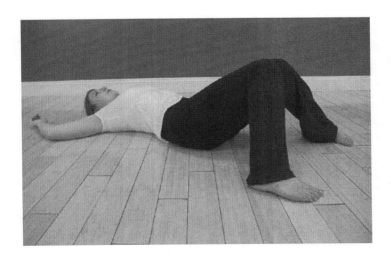

## 12. Diaphragmatic Breathing

Lie down on your back with knees bent, soles flat on the ground, feet hip distance apart. Relax your shoulders, bring the palm of the

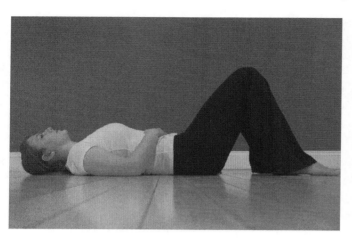

right hand to the navel. Shift your attention to the navel. As you exhale mentally observe your navel going down toward the spine. Inhale deep and slowly, mentally observe your navel rising smoothly. Again, exhale, mentally notice your navel falling; inhale, notice your navel raising. Repeat several times. At the end of each exhalation, gently squeeze your navel toward the spine. Relax the abdominal muscles

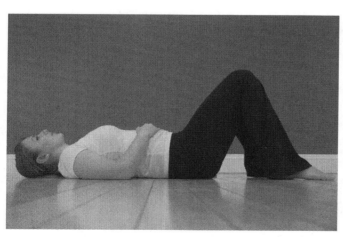

and repeat this smooth conscious abdominal breathing for 3 to 5 mins. Maintain your attention on the navel, relax shoulders and face.

## 13. Press Leg Towards Abdomen/Fetus Pose

Lie down on your back with knees bent, soles on the ground, feet

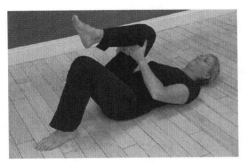

parallel and hip distance apart. Exhale, bring your right thigh to the chest, clasp your hands behind it and gently press the thigh towards you. Inhale, release the pressure. Exhale and again gently press the thigh towards

your abdomen. After several breaths, unclasp the hands, exhale and lower the foot back to the ground. Repeat with the left leg. Now, bring both legs to the chest, embrace and gently press them towards the chest as

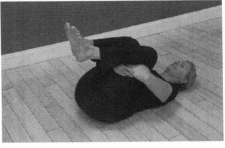

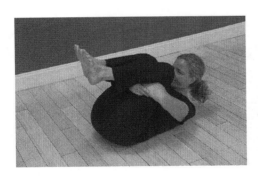

you inhale and exhale. After a few breaths, keep the gentle pressure on the thighs, inhale and lift the head towards the knees; exhale bring your head back down to the ground. Repeat three times and release the pressure.

72

## 14. Cat Pose

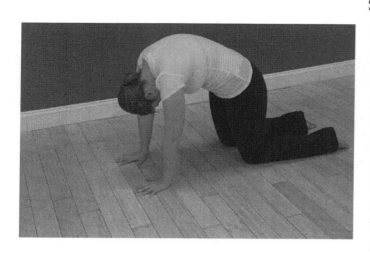

Start in a table position, hands underneath the shoulders, knees underneath the hips. As you exhale, tuck your tailbone under, and gradually round your middle back and drop your head. Inhale, slowly lift your tailbone, curve your back in the other direction and look up. Repeat several times moving slowly and steadily. Synchronize breath and the motion.

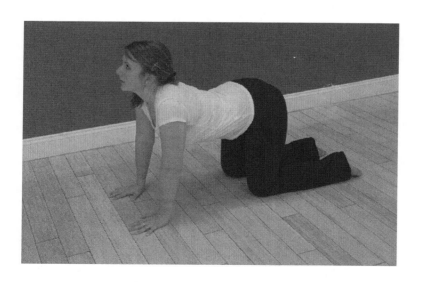

## 15. Half Dog Variation

Start in a table position, hands underneath the shoulders, knees underneath the hips. Lower your forearms to the ground, keep

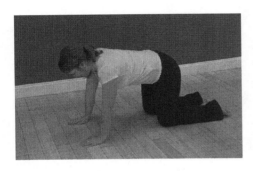

elbows underneath your shoulders and forearms parallel to each other. Place your right hand behind your left elbow. Slide your left arm away from you straightening out this arm. Inhale, gently press your hips back and away from you; exhale slowly lower your forehead on or towards the ground. Hold this position for several breaths focusing on abdominal breathing. Come back to the table position and repeat on the other side.

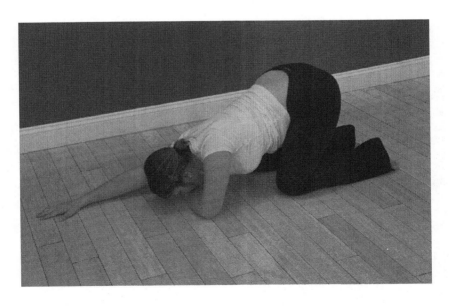

## 16. Downward Facing Dog / Table

Start in a table position, hands underneath the shoulders, knees

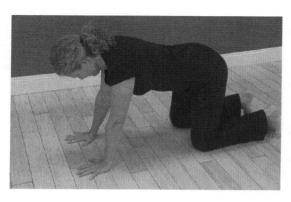

underneath the hips. Inhale and curl your toes under. Exhale, press your palms into the ground, lift your hips into downward dog. Inhale, come back to table pose. Repeat for a few times dog and table alternately. Pause in the dog position and move your heels up and down alternately for several times, as if you were walking in place. Stop the motion, keep feet shoulder width apart and parallel to each other, press both heels on or towards the ground; gently press hips upward, as you softly press

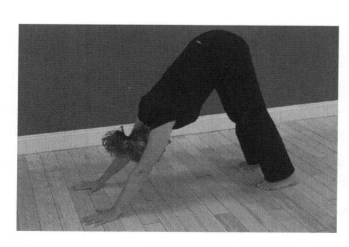

your chest towards the thighs. Relax your head and neck. Look at your knees. Hold for a few breaths. Walk your hands to the feet and slowly lift the spine. Stand up.

## 17. Wood Chopper

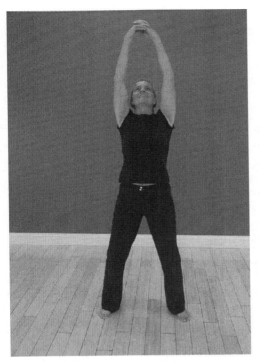

Stand with feet shoulder distance apart and knees slightly bent. Bend forward from the hips, clasp your hands close to the floor as if you were holding an axe. As you inhale slowly raise both arms overhead. Gaze at the hands as you raise the arms. Pause. Exhale with a strong sigh (HA sound) and fold forward keeping your knees bent. Allow your hands and arms to swing down. Re-clasp your hands, keep your knees slightly bent and lift again.

Repeat several times. Imagine that you are chopping wood - holding an axe in your hand as you lift the arms up and chopping the wood with the axe as you fold forward.

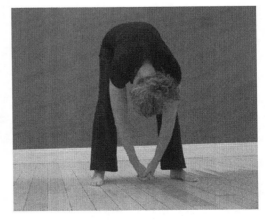

## 18. Triangle (beginners and advanced)

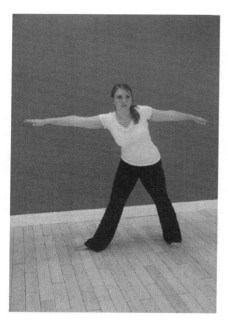

Separate your feet about three feet apart. Turn your right foot to a ninety degree angle. Turn left foot at a slight angle inward toward the right. Inhale and bring both arms at shoulder height. Exhale and lean your trunk to the right. Inhale, engage the right knee. As you exhale, lean a little more to the right and tilt the arms. Right arm lands on right leg and left arms points to the ceiling. Slowly, look down at the right foot. Notice where your right arm naturally meets the right leg.

Inhale, tuck your tailbone under and slowly look up at the right hand pointing to the ceiling. Exhale, upper chest forward, left shoulder slightly back. Make sure both shoulders remain in line with each other. If the left shoulder starts to fold forward bring your right hand higher into the right leg until your shoulders are in line with each other. The crown of the head is reaching directly out to the right. Hold this position for a few breaths.

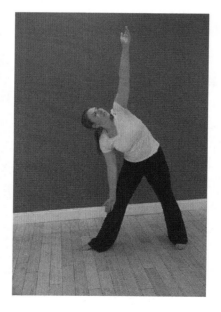

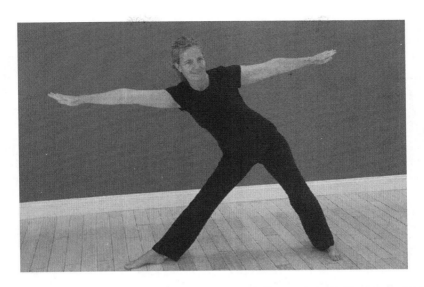

When you are ready to come out of the pose, inhale, press both feet into the ground, lift your torso and bring both arms directly out to your sides. Exhale and lower your arms. Repeat on the other side turning your left foot out to a ninety degree angle and your right foot at a slight angle inward toward the left.

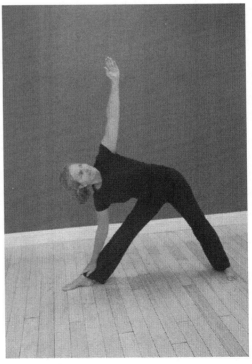

## 19. Revolved Triangle

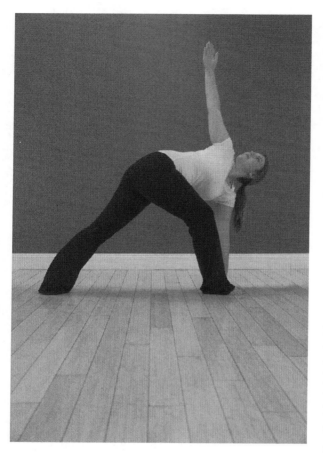

Come into the triangle position with right foot facing toward the right. Lower both arms and bring the palms of the hands on the floor by your right foot. Bend the right knee as much you need for the hands to reach the floor. Press the left hand on the floor and slowly lift your right arm, as you turn your head look up at the right hand pointing up, fingertips reaching up towards the ceiling. Hold this position for a few breaths. To come out of the pose return to the triangle, lower the right hand to the floor, lift the left arm and bring the right hand to the right leg. Come back into the triangle position. As you inhale, press both feet into the ground, raise your torso up, bring both arms directly out to your sides, exhale and bring the arms down by your sides.

## 20. Advanced Breathing

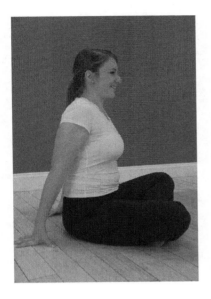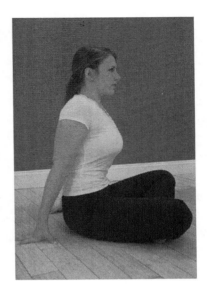

Sit upright in a cross legged position. Head facing forward with your chin parallel to the ground. Bring the right hand to the navel and practice your abdominal breathing. Exhale, navel in toward your spine. Relax your abdominal muscles. Inhale, breathe deeply and slowly and notice your belly moving forward. Exhale, and gently bring your navel toward the spine. Repeat several times to warm up the diaphragm muscle.

Now, inhale deeply into the lower abdomen, and mentally observe your navel moving forward. Exhale, draw your navel in toward your spine and at the end of this exhalation, gradually squeeze the abdomen, perineum, sphincter and anal muscles. Hold the squeeze, without air and bring your belly in and up. Hold for a few seconds and relax the diaphragm and abdomen. Repeat this breathing twice more. You can also practice the advanced breathing lying down on the floor, if more comfortable.

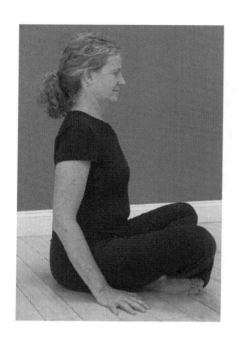
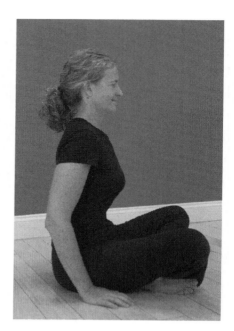

## 21. Knees and Elbows Motion

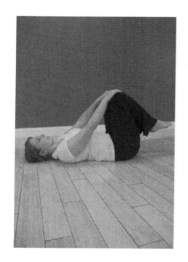

Lie down on your back with knees bent and feet off the floor. Place the right and left hand on the top of the knees, fingertips pointing toward the feet. Exhale and as you inhale gradually straighten both arms out and move knees away from you. Exhale, bring your knees toward your chest. Synchronize breath and motion. Repeat several times. Feel the gentle massage on the lower back as you do the motion.

Now, inhale and straighten both arms out, knees away from you and also bring legs up with soles toward the ceiling (legs at a right angle to the torso). Now, bring the hands behind your thighs. Exhale, bend the knees and bring your legs back toward the chest. Repeat several times and at the end lower the soles to the ground.

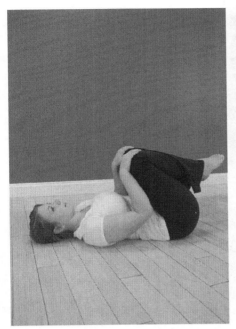
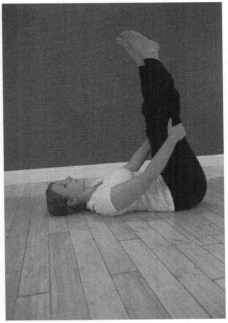

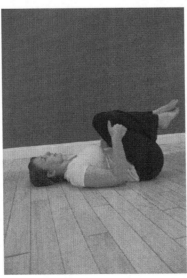

## 22. **Reclined Twist**

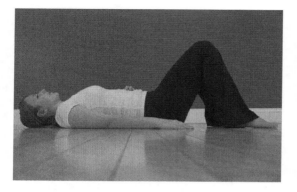

Lie down on your back with arms by your sides and away from you. Bend your knees, soles flat on the ground; keep feet and knees together. Inhale deeply and as you exhale lower both knees to the left,

left thigh touches the ground. The right leg rests on top of the left. Momentarily, hold breath and motion. Inhale and raise both knees back up. Exhale and lower the knees to the right; right thigh touches the floor.

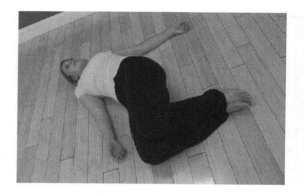

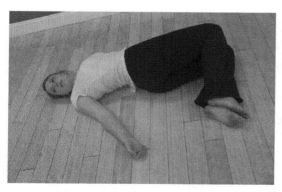

Hold briefly. Inhale and raise both knees back up. Repeat the motion to the left and to the right several times, synchronize both breath and motion.

## 23. Final Relaxation - *Shavasana*

Lie on your back with arms by your sides and slightly away from you, palms facing up; legs slightly apart. Relax your shoulders. Allow your breathing to become natural. Slowly move your head

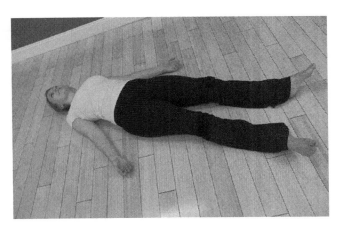

from side to side, almost as if you were not doing it. Do it calmly and passively. Allow your head to come back to the center and pause. Gently, close your eyes. Relax your face and let your eyes soften. Now, there is nothing else for you to do or to undo, nothing for you to force or to accomplish. Relaxation is only a feeling. Abandon your entire body on the floor. As you relax more, bring your attention inside, to the vast ocean of peace and harmony that is already within. Nothing can disturb you right now. Feel the calm that surfaces the body. Soak in these waves of peace. The more you relax, the more you restore. Remain in this position for at least 10 minutes.

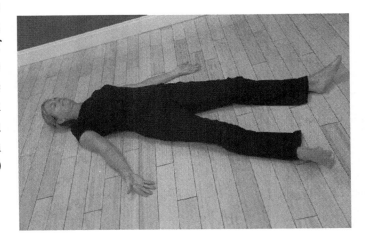

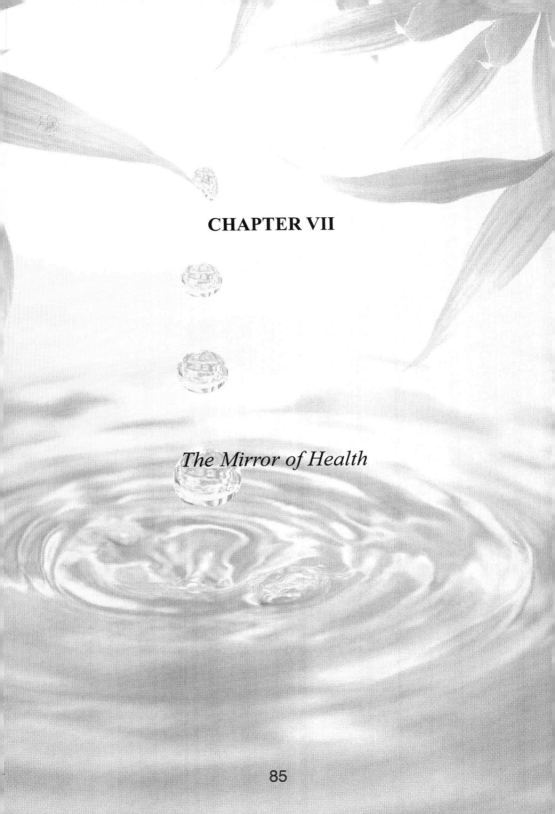

# CHAPTER VII

*The Mirror of Health*

Today, it appears that we are finding ways to slow down the aging process. Now, we can look younger using new technology and advanced creams. We are trying to smooth wrinkles out, to make the face look more youthful. It seems we are defeating the aging process.

But not so fast! This is just the outward appearance. It is simply an illusion. While the outside pretends to look younger, everything inside the body is decaying. Cellular activity is slowing down, tissues and functions are getting worn out and deteriorating over time. The external appearance cannot change the internal decline.

We still have the same diseases of any old person in the past or even worse. New diseases have developed because of our fast paced environment, depleted food, polluted water and air, over working, over medication and myriad other causes.

Diseases are often addressed by amazing advancements in science that create better or stronger medicines. But, we must also recognize that these medicines usually do not effectively address the root cause of the disease and may create serious side effects.

How many people die because of overdoses of what is supposed to cure them? How many people take antibiotics and have allergic reactions? How many people go through surgery and find the result worse than their original symptoms? How many of us suffer from medical errors? How many of us are taking medicines that solve a problem and create another one, sometimes even worse?

We must recognize the effort of our researchers and scholars. They are doing their best, investing their lives for the common good. Significant progress has been achieved. But, perhaps we are blind to the fact that science cannot prevent diseases from creeping in and cannot efficiently solve them. We may recognize that there is a disconnection in our health issues, that perhaps something is missing and that there is room for improvement.

But, how? Maybe the direction for improvement is totally different than expected. We need to think out of the box. Maybe things are simpler than previously thought and we all can have a more dignified and healthier life until the end of our journey.

## PROBLEM AND SOLUTION

Invariably, if there is a problem, there is a solution. Yoga believes that both problem and solution are together.

This Yoga concept - where the problem is, there also lies the solution - can radically change the way we perceive our challenges. It means that when a problem emerges we need to look as closely as possible at it, because therein lies the solution. **Problem and solution are always together**.

When we look far for the resolution of any problem, we are doomed to fail, according to this ancient concept. When we move away from the problem, we only find palliatives, which really are not the solution.

The fact that sometimes it is hard or takes a long time to find the solution does not mean the solution does not exist. It simply means that, probably, we are not looking in the right direction. Maybe the solution is so simple, so close to the problem, we cannot see it.

For instance, we all have cancer cells. The immune function of the Lymphatic System is in charge of neutralizing and expelling them, which it does, most of the time. Sometimes it does not.

We may wonder: why does cancer hit all types of people even those that do have a heathy life style? If having a good diet and proper exercise would keep cancer away, then healthy, conscientious people should not have this disease. But, this is not our reality - all types of people are hit by this disease.

Maybe the answer to this enigma is so simple and so close to us that we are unable to see it. How about if we look for answers in the areas closest to the problem?

So, if cancer does not have an easy solution and this disease essentially is an immune system deficiency, the only solution is to take a closer look at the immune function of the Lymphatic System and understand how to strengthen it.

This system is the foundation of health for all other systems of the body, since it permeates, nourishes and cleans them. As a result, it also determines conditions in all of them. At the same time the Lymphatic System is part of the immune system, which is in charge of getting rid of cancer cells.

Probably, a moving lymph is the answer to this riddle. Probably, avoiding lymph stagnation is the solution we were looking for. Probably, ensuring the activation and renewal of the "water of life" is all that is necessary to avoid and resolve many health conditions.

The Lymphatic System is the septic system, the nourisher and also the defender of all other bodily systems. A continuous lymph flow assures the removal of toxins and debris while it prevents bacteria and waste stagnation. Consequently, cell nourishment becomes more efficient, tissue repair is accelerated and the lymph nodes - not overloaded by debris - are able to quickly and more effectively respond to invaders with an increasing production of lymphocytes. So, the immune response also becomes more powerful.

A moving lymph stream becomes the effective solution for many bodily unpleasant conditions. We are in charge of our own health. Nobody else is. It is important to be proactive, to keep the lymph fluid moving and use Lymphatic Yoga practice as a preventative method and hit the disease before it arrives and not after the problem is already manifested.

The care of the Lymphatic System, along with proper diet and proper sleep is a simple and natural solution. This is the way the body was designed to work, naturally.

Now is the time to return to the basis and origin of our own being to recharge and restore in the "water of life" within. Now is the time to take care of ourselves to be able to take care of others. To live in harmony it is necessary to return to our roots, to return to the "water of life" that we all came from and that is now within us represented by the Lymphatic System, the mirror of our health.

# Reference

(1) Foldi M., Foldi E., "Foldi's Textbook of Lymphology" , Chapter 3 by Rautenfeld D.B. and Schacht V., Elsevier, 2006 (2nd Edition)

(2) Wittlinger G., Wittlinger H., "Textbook of Dr. Vodder's Manual Lymph Drainage", Thieme, 2004: 16-17.

(3) Foldi M., R. StroBenreuther, "Foundations of Manual Lymph Drainage", Elsevier, 2003: 6-7

(4) Chikly, B, "Silent Waves: Theory and Practice of Lymph Drainage Therapy", International Health & Healing Inc, 2004, 2nd Ed.: 35

(5) Foldi M., Foldi E., "Foldi's Textbook of Lymphology" , Chapter 4 by M. Foldi and E. Foldi, Elsevier, 2006, 2nd Ed.: 193

(6) Foldi M., Foldi E., "Foldi's Textbook of Lymphology" , Chapter 4 by M. Foldi and E. Foldi, Elsevier, 2006, 2nd Ed.: 203

(7) Foldi M., R. StroBenreuther, "Foundations of Manual Lymph Drainage", Elsevier, 2003: 3

(8) Kasseroller R., "Compendium of Dr. Vodder's Manual Lymph Drainage", Haug, 1998: 49

(9) Foldi M., R. StroBenreuther, "Foundations of Manual Lymph Drainage", Elsevier, 2003: 32-33

(10)Kasseroller R., "Compendium of Dr. Vodder's Manual Lymph Drainage", Haug, 1998: 49

(11)Klose G., Francis K., "LTCC - Lymphedema Therapy Certification Course" manual, Klose Training & Consulting, 2010

(12)Sappey, Ph. C., "Traite' D'Anatomie Descriptive" - 2nd volume, 1868, 12th Ed.:796-797; Foldi M., Foldi E., "Foldi's Textbook of Lymphology" , Chapter 1 by S. Kubick and O.Kretz, Elsevier, 2006, 2nd Ed.: 9

(13)Foldi M., R. StroBenreuther, "Foundations of Manual Lymph Drainage", Elsevier, 2003: 8

(14)Klose G., Francis K., "LTCC - Lymphedema Therapy Certification Course" manual, Klose Training & Consulting, 2010

(15)"Foldi's Textbook of Lymphology" , Chapter 1 by S. Kubick and O.Kretz, Elsevier, 2006, 2nd Ed.: 9; Kasseroller R., "Compendium of Dr. Vodder's Manual Lymph Drainage", Haug, 1998: 52

(16)Klose G., Francis K., "LTCC - Lymphedema Therapy Certification Course", Klose Training & Consulting, 2010

(17)Foldi M., Foldi E., "Foldi's Textbook of Lymphology", Chapter 4 by M. Foldi and E. Foldi, Elsevier, 2006, 2nd Ed.

(18)Ker, Than, National Geographic Magazine, published February 16, 2010.

# Bibliography

**Works on Yoga**

1.Desikashar, T.K.S., *Yoga Entretien Sur la Theorie et la Pratique*, Viniyoga, Paris, 1982.

2.Dechanet, J.M., O.S.B., *Yoga in Ten Lessons,* Cornerstone Library, N.York, 1973

3.Kerneiz, C., *Le Yoga de L'Occident,* Ed. Belenos, Quebec, 2002.

4.Kuvalayananda, Swami, *Asanas,* Cultrix, S.Paulo, 1993

5.Lysebeth, Andre Van , *Yoga Self-Taught*, Weiser, N. York, 1999.

6.Lysebeth, Andre Van, *Ma Seance de Yoga*, Flamarion, France, 1977.

7.Lysebeth, Van Lysebeth, *Pranayama La Dynamique du Souffle*, Flamarion, France, 1971.

8.Lysebeth, Andre Van, *Aperfeicoando o Meu Yoga*, C.L.B., Lisboa, 1979.

9.Miranda, Caio, *A Libertacao pelo Yoga*, NAP, Rio de Janeiro, 1960.

10.Ramacharaka, *Science of Breath*, Yogi Publication Society, Chicago, 1905.

11.Saraswati, Swami Satyananda, *Asana Pranayama Mudra Bandha*, Bihar School of Yoga, India, 1999.

12.Sivananda, *Practice of Yoga*, Divine Life Society, India, 1984.

13.Sivananda, *A Ciencia do Pranayama,* Ed. Pensamento*, S.Paulo, 1993.*

14.Sivananda Yoga Center, *The Sivananda Companion to Yoga,* Simon & Schuster, 1983.

15. Taimni, I.K., *The Science of Yoga,* A Quest Book, Madras/London, 1986

16.Vishnu-Devananda, Swami, *The Complete Illustrated Book of Yoga*, Harmony Books, N.York, 1988

17.Yesudian S. & Haich E., *Yoga and Health,* Allen and Unwin, 1966.

## About the Author

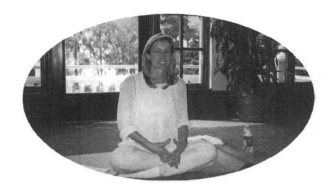

Edely L. Wallace, BA, E-RYT, CDT is a Yoga master who studied with Andre Van Lysebeth in Belgium and trained in the US and Brazil in several yoga traditions. In 2003 she founded the "Yogamatrix Studio" in Orlando, FL and is presently the studio's Executive Director.

She is a former Executive Board Member (2002-2005) of "Yoga Alliance" and was the Yoga Consultant for the Orange County Public School in Orlando, FL (1999-2003). She has taught Yoga for Florida Hospital Celebration Health and Osceola Regional Hospital. Edely has been featured in several TV shows including "Daily Buzz" and "Morning News" at Fox 35. She writes for local magazines about Yoga and health.

Since 2000, she has trained over 300 Yoga Teachers. In 2004, she released a DVD entitled "Yoga For Stress Relief". She has taught Yoga workshops and retreats nationally and internationally. In 2010, she began teaching the unique "Lymphatic Yoga" class, which incorporates her vast knowledge of Yoga and the Lymphatic System into a practical application for everyone.

She was first exposed to Yoga after a grave accident that left her bedridden for several years in the 1980s. Her intense study of Yoga techniques helped in her recovery. Over 20 years ago, she began studying lymphatic drainage therapy. After many years of combining Yoga and lymphatic drainage in her personal yoga practice, Edely is now ready to release her findings and share the results with others. This is a new method that holds the key to health, preventative care and rejuvenation, in a natural way.

Edely studied Mathematics at the university (FAFI) in Brazil and later taught Math at the junior High School level. After coming to the US, se attended the University of Central FL (UCF) and received a B.A. in Philosophy. Edely is a Massage Therapist and is certified as a Lymph Therapist (CDT - Complete Decongestive Therapy) by the renowned "Foldi Clinic" in Hinterzarten, Germany.


www.yogamatrixstudio.com

Made in the USA
Middletown, DE
20 October 2015